Contents

INTRODUCTION 4

CHAPTER ONE 5

WHAT IS OXALATE? 5

How does this happen and why is it a problem? 5

Protections from oxalate 7

CHAPTER TWO 10

LOW OXALATE DIET RECIPES 10

BREAKFAST: 10

Cottage Cheese Pancakes 10

No-Bake Low Oxalate Protein Bars 11

Paleo Pancakes 14

BREAD AND MUFFINS: 15

Sunflower Spice Paleo Quick Bread 15

Coconut Flour Banana Bread 17

Coconut Flour Zucchini Bread 19

DESSERTS: 20

Ginger Pumpkin Custard 20

Holiday Baked Apples 22

Best Banana Ice Cream 24

Dips and Appetizers: 26

Black-Eye Pea Fritters (Akara) 26

Dash of salt 26

Medium Oxalate Hummus 30

MAIN DISHES:... 32

Broccoli Beef... 32

Chicken Enchiladas Verde 33

Verde Sauce.. 35

French Beef Stew 36

Low Oxalate Sunbutter Burgers.......................... 39

Beverages.. 41

Banana Blueberry Dairy-Free Milkshakes 41

Hot Chocolate Steamer 42

MAIN DISHES (VEGETARIAN):................................ 43

Jamaican Rice and Peas................................ 45

Kohlrabi Risotto 46

Vegan Stuffed Red Peppers.............................. 49

SALADS:.. 51

Apple Pineapple Salad 51

Cilantro Lime Slaw 53

Avocado Egg Salad 54

OTHER RECIPES.. 56

Sarah's Applesauce 56

Pretzel Turtles 57

Smooth Sweet Tea 58

Sauteed Apples.. 59

Delicious Ham and Potato Soup 61

Tasty Collard Greens 63

Sausage Stuffed Jalapenos 65

Rosemary Roasted Turkey....................................... 67

Best Lemonade Ever 69

Luscious Slush Punch 70

Homestyle Turkey, the Michigander Way............ 73

Big Al's K.C. Bar-B-Q Sauce 74

Southern Pimento Cheese....................................... 76

Guacamole 78

Grilled Asparagus.. 79

Grilled Marinated Shrimp....................................... 81

Jamie's Sweet and Easy Corn on the Cob............. 83

Roasted Rack of Lamb.. 84

Roasted Rack of Lamb.. 86

Amish White Bread 86

Low oxalate snacks 88

BLT Wraps 91

Fruit salad... 92

Low oxalate breakfast ideas.................................... 92

Banana Muffins 92

Banana smoothie.. 94

CONCLUSION.. 95

INTRODUCTION

Oxalate is a very simple sort of molecule. It links up with calcium and crystallizes under some conditions, including when it encounters damaged tissues. The crystals formed this way can be quite irritating and painful to tissues where they cause or increase inflammation. These crystals can be especially painful if they lodge themselves in places where they get in the way of the movement of other things through tight places.

The idea of a low-oxalate diet is confusing. Restricting nutritious foods unnecessarily is stressful it's already hard enough to know how to eat healthy. And while high-oxalate foods can contribute to kidney stone formation in some people, the benefits of their nutritional profile generally outweigh the risks, particularly when you take the preventative measures outlined above.

Use these tips as inspiration to hydrate more, seek out calcium-rich foods, and make nutritious food combinations. And as always, consult with your healthcare provider about any health concerns, and try to enjoy the least restrictive diet possible made up of real, whole foods.

CHAPTER ONE

WHAT IS OXALATE?

Oxalate is present in a lot of plants and fruit that we eat. It is especially high in almost all seeds and nuts, but in some more than others. Ordinarily, the gut won't absorb much of the oxalate from the diet because most of the oxalate will be metabolized by the flora or just leave the body with the stool. Under other conditions, such as when there is gut inflammation, a lot of dietary oxalate is absorbed. The difference can be as great as going from 1-2% of the dietary oxalate absorbed to as high as 50%.

Over absorption of oxalate will also occur when the tight junctions between intestinal cells open up and let molecules pass to the other side going between the cells. This condition, called the "leaky gut", may happen during illness, or when cells in the gut die, leaving gaps, and may bring with it allergies to foods. This condition is similar to when the bladder has open junctions called the "leaky bladder", or when the blood brain barrier is compromised. The colon may also absorb too much oxalate when small bowel function is compromised by surgery, by poor pancreatic function, and/or by fat maldigestion.

How does this happen and why is it a problem?

When substances move to the blood from the gut by slipping around intestinal cells, they bypass the regulation that is present when these same substances move across through the inside of these cells. Intestinal cells can control the quantity that crosses. They do this by regulating the number of transporters or carriers that span the cell membrane and allow that particular substance into the cell. After a substance crosses the cell to the blood side, it can leave the cell to join the blood using a different set of transporters that are on the blood or "exit" side. These transporters are very specific for particular chemicals or nutrients.

Because intestinal cells control admission and exit from both the gut and blood side, that's why the body can send signals to these cells instructing them whether to absorb more or absorb less of a substance from food. So cells can erect barriers, if you will, to prevent too much of a substance to cross, and this regulation can protect us.

Unfortunately, the body loses that regulation when substances are absorbed through the leaky junctions between cells. Oxalate is just one of the unfortunate substances where unregulated absorption is a problem. At least now we know about oxalate, but other things in food may also be a problem, like gluten, and for some, casein, or allergenic foods.

Whenever more oxalate is absorbed like this, the result is increased levels of oxalate in blood and urine and in tissues. More of it stays in the bone than anywhere, but it also goes into blood vessels, and glands, and secretory organs and even the spleen and heart. It can even get into the brain, most likely the parts of the brain that regulate hormones.

Our bodies can also make oxalate

Eating foods high in oxalate is not the only way for oxalate to get high in cells and blood. Our bodies make oxalate on their own, especially when certain enzymes aren't balanced in their activity because of genetic differences or because someone has deficiencies in enzyme cofactors like vitamin B6, magnesium or thiamine. Oxalate also can be generated in the body when someone is getting high doses of vitamin C or consuming high levels of fructose.

Protections from oxalate

Normally, when oxalate travels through the gut, it may encounter particular species of bacteria which will digest it and turn it into something else that isn't so irritating and harmful. This system of microbial digestion of oxalate may be why the body seems to purposefully route excess oxalate from the rest of the body to the gut for disposal. Unfortunately, the very microbes we need to do this digesting of oxalate for us are subject to being killed by antibiotics in common use. Even if there was no exposure to antibiotics, these microbes might not have colonized in very young children. The main oxalate degrading bacteria, oxalobacter formigenes, does not tend to be present in breastmilk, but scientists think it must be picked up gradually from the environment.

Lactobacillus acidophilus deprived of its usual food, may be able to "eat" oxalate, but too much oxalate in its diet may kill it off. This may explain why certain people have great difficulty colonizing lactobacillus acidophilus, despite constant use of probiotics containing it.

Fortunately, a probiotic formulation of a bacteria called oxalobacter formigenes is under development as a drug for patients with hyperoxaluria and related conditions, and it is currently in clinical trials, but may not be available until 2012 or 2013.

Whole foods considered high in oxalates include:

Fruits: berries, figs, kiwis, purple grapes

Vegetables: spinach, Swiss chard, leeks, okra, rhubarb, beets

Nuts, seeds, and grains: almonds, cashews, peanuts, soy, wheat bran, wheat germ, quinoa, chocolate, cocoa

Tea

So just how worried should you be and should you embrace a low-oxalate diet? Should you strike these foods from your menu entirely? Or is there a way to work around oxalates? Here's what you need to know.

Cottage Cheese Pancakes

4 eggs, beaten

1 cup cottage cheese

1/2 C sweet rice flour (mochi) or 1/4 C coconut flour

Dash salt

1/2 teaspoon baking soda (optional)

coconut oil, butter or ghee for frying

Mix eggs, cottage cheese, flour and salt in a bowl with a spout if possible. Heat about ½ tablespoon oil in a skillet over medium heat until it's hot enough to sizzle. Pour pancake batter into the skillet in 1/3 to 1/2 cup portions. Cook until bubbles start to form on top of the pancakes and the underneath in golden brown (about 3 or 4 minutes). Flip the pancakes once and cook another 1-2 minutes. Serve cottage cheese pancakes with the traditional butter and syrup, or try honey, jam, fresh fruit, sour cream or plain yogurt mixed with a little syrup.

Yeild: 6-8 pancakes (recipe easily halves, doubles or triples)

1 ½ cups of GF rolled oats

½ cup of ground flax seed

1 cup of whey protein powder (or use rice protein, egg white protein or pea protein powder)

½ cup of flaked coconut (unsweetened)

¾ cup of raisins (or dried cherries, dried apples or dried blueberries)

2 tablespoons of pumpkin seeds

½ cup of honey (or half a dropper of liquid)

½ cup plus 2 tablespoons of Sunbutter (or other low oxalate sunflower seed spread)

3-4 tablespoons of butter or coconut oil

2 teaspoons of vanilla extract

1-3 tablespoons of water

Combine the oats, flax seed, protein powder, coconut, raisins and pumpkin seeds in a bowl and mix well. Put the honey, Sunbutter, butter and vanilla in a separate glass or ceramic dish and microwave on high for about 30 – 45 seconds until the butter is melted and the Sunbutter is gooey. Stir the Sunbutter mixture until it is well combined.

Add the Sunbutter mixture and the oat mixture and stir until the oats are well coated. It should have a crumbly, somewhat dry texture that barely holds together when you press it (like the oatmeal topping of an apple crisp). Add the water a half tablespoon at a time, stirring well each time, until you get a mixture that will hold together more like playdough (still a little dry but could be rolled into one big ball that would stay together). It usually takes about 2 tablespoons water.

Press the oat mixture into a 9 X 9 inch baking dish OR other convenient dish with about the same dimensions (you could press it directly into a convenient-sized Tupperware). I often use a Pyrex glass baking dish with a plastic lid. For easy removal, line the bottom of the pan with plastic wrap plus enough to double back over the top as a cover after you've pressed the oat mixture into it. Put the dish into the refrigerator and let chill overnight or for at least four hours. Cut into 18 bars (4.5 x 1 inch each). Transfer into an air tight container (or wrap in the plastic wrap) and keep refrigerated for up to two weeks (Maybe three? I've never had them that long, but there's nothing in here that doesn't keep a long time in the refrigerator).

Makes 18 bars.

4 eggs

1 tablespoon of coconut milk or water

1/2 dropper of liquid stevia or a teaspoon honey (optional)

1/4 teaspoon of baking soda (optional)

1/4 cup of coconut flour

Coconut oil or butter for cooking (we use pastured butter)

Put all ingredients (except the oil) in the blender and blend until smooth (make sure you put the coconut flour in last or in will turn into cement in the bottom of your blender!). Let sit for two or three minutes to thicken up (A fun property of coconut flour is all the fiber which slowly absorbs liquid as it sits. If it gets too thick add a little more water). Pour pancakes onto a hot, oiled griddle or skillet and cook until edges are brown and you start to see bubbles (smaller pancakes are much easier to flip). Flip pancake and continue cooking until golden brown on both sides. Serve hot with fresh fruit, low oxalate spreadable fruit (we love these with home-made apple butter), maple syrup, sunflower butter, butter or plain yogurt (if you do dairy). You can also make a yummy fruit syrup by simply pureeing blueberries or strawberries in the blender with a little liquid stevia. These pancakes are great cold as a snack or lunchbox stuffer the next day– plain or with sunflower butter, butter, or low oxalate spreadable fruit. This recipe also works as a waffle recipe!

Makes 6-8 pancakes. Recipe doubles easily if you have a large blender!

Note: If you are cooking for a crowd, set your oven to 150 degrees and put a cookie sheet on the top rack which you've set in the middle of the oven to make it easy to reach in. Put pancakes on the cookie sheet as they come off the griddle to keep them warm and yummy until you have enough to serve.

BREAD AND MUFFINS:
Sunflower Spice Paleo Quick Bread
1/2 cup of Sunbutter

2 eggs

1/4 cup of honey (or 2 T honey, plus a half dropper liquid Stevia)

1 teaspoon of vanilla extract

1/2 – 1 tablespoon of lemon juice (optional, see warning)

1/4 teaspoon of baking soda

pinch of Celtic sea salt

1/2 teaspoon of nutmeg

1/4 teaspoon of cardamom

1/4 teaspoon of cinnamon (optional)

Preheat the oven to 325 degrees.   Place the Sunbutter in a bowl and mix with a hand mixer until the Sunbutter is really creamy. Add the eggs, honey, vanilla and mix a little more. Add the baking soda, salt, nutmeg, cardamom and cinnamon and mix until thoroughly blended. Put in a greased 8 x 8 ceramic or Pyrex baking dish and bake at 325 degrees for about 14 minutes.

Makes 12 small squares.

Note: It's hard to get the baking soda to mix evenly in this recipe since you don't have a flour to mix your baking soda into before adding the wet ingredients. It works best for me to mix the baking soda with the spices and salt, then slowly sprinkle the dry ingredients over the wet ingredients with a little mixing in between.

Warning: (added on 4/19/2012) As one of my readers pointed out in the comments below, I forgot to warn you that the chlorogenic acid in sunflower seeds reacts with baking soda and turns green as your bread cools. Yes, that's right. If you do not eat all of this bread within about three hours you too will have green bread, especially if you looked at my recipe and thought "No way is 1/4 teaspoon baking soda going to be enough" and put in 1/2 teaspoon instead. Might be fun on St. Patrick's Day! Anyway, there are two ways to keep your bread from turning green. You may reduce the baking soda to about 1/8 teaspoon, but it won't rise very well. You may also add about a 1/2 – 1 tablespoon lemon juice, which isn't bad.

Low Oxalate Info: Sunbutter (6.1 mg. oxalate per 2 tablespoon), nutmeg (9.4 mg. per teaspoon) and 1/4 teaspoon cinnamon (9.5 mg. per 1/4 teaspoon) are medium oxalate ingredients. All other ingredients are very low oxalate. Sunflower Spice Paleo Quick Bread has about 4.6 mg. oxalate per serving when made without the cinnamon or 5.5 mg. oxalate per serving when made with the cinnamon.

Coconut Flour Banana Bread

Modified by Heidi Stallman from a recipe by Leanne Vogel.

4 eggs

3/4 cup of mashed banana (2-3 fresh or frozen bananas)

1/4 cup of coconut oil, melted

1/4 cup of low oxalate coconut milk (I use Natural Value coconut milk)

2 tbsp of unpasteurized honey (or a dropper full of liquid Stevia)

1/2 tsp of pure vanilla extract

1/4 tsp of cinnamon extract or cinnamon oil* (optional – please see low oxalate info below)

1/2 cup of coconut flour

1/2 tsp of gluten-free baking soda

Preheat oven to 350 degrees and line an 8 x 4-inch loaf pan with parchment paper across both sides for easy lifting OR grease pan well (I use coconut oil spray). Set aside. Combine eggs, bananas, coconut milk, oil, honey, vanilla extract and cinnamon extract in a large bowl with an electric mixer (using a mixer gives this bread an airier texture than mixing by hand). Whisk coconut flour and baking soda in a small bowl. Once mixed, slowly add the dry ingredients to the wet mixture and mix until smooth (Warning: if you add it all at once you might get "coconut flour cement!") Pour batter into prepared loaf pan and bake in preheated oven for 40-45 minutes or until toothpick inserted comes out clean. Remove from the oven and allow to cool for 5 minutes. Remove from pan and allow to cool on a cooling rack for 20 -4o minutes before slicing and serving. My family likes to eat this bread warm with butter, but you might also like it plain or topped with coconut oil or sunflower seed butter.

Makes 10 – 12 slices.

Coconut Flour Zucchini Bread

4 eggs

1/4 cup of coconut oil, melted

1 tsp of pure vanilla extract

1/4 cup of low oxalate coconut milk (I use Natural Value coconut milk)

1/2 cup of coconut flour

1/2 tsp of gluten-free baking soda

1/4 tsp. of salt

1/2 tsp of cardamom (optional)

1/2 – 1 teaspoon of Now Organic Stevia Powder

1 cup of shredded zucchini (or yellow summer squash), water squeezed out

Preheat oven to 350 degrees and line an 8 x 4-inch loaf pan with parchment paper across both sides for easy lifting OR grease pan well (I use coconut oil spray or ghee). Set aside. Combine eggs, oil, coconut milk and vanilla extract in a large bowl with an electric mixer (using a mixer or blender gives this bread an airier texture than mixing by hand). Whisk coconut flour, baking soda, salt, cardamom and Stevia powder in a small bowl. Once mixed, slowly add the dry ingredients to the wet mixture and mix until smooth (Warning: if you add it all at once you might get "coconut flour cement) Add the shredded zucchini and mix well (use your hand to squeeze it out over the sink before you throw it in). Pour batter into prepared loaf pan and bake in preheated oven for 40-45 minutes or until toothpick inserted comes out clean. Remove from the oven and allow to cool for 5 minutes. Remove from pan and allow to cool on a cooling rack for 20 -4o minutes before slicing and serving. I personally prefer this bread plain and cold out of the fridge, but you may enjoy yours topped with butter, coconut oil, cream cheese or sunflower seed butter.

Makes 10 – 12 slices.

Ginger Pumpkin Custard

2 cups pumpkin puree (see note on how to bake a pumpkin)

3 eggs

3/4 cup cream, half and half or coconut milk*

1/4 – 1/2 cup honey

1 tablespoon of raw ginger, minced or grated (I use a garlic press to mince the ginger)

1 teaspoon of nutmeg

1 teaspoon of vanilla extract (optional)

Dash salt

Preheat oven to 325 degrees. Put all the ingredients in bowl and stir until well mixed. Turn into a greased 8 x 8 baking dish or pie plate (see note on baking dishes). Bake for about 40-45 minutes until the center is set. Serve warm or cold (we like it cold). If serving as a desert (higher sugar version) you may want to add a dollop of whipped cream. If serving as breakfast or side dish (lower sugar version), you may want to add a dollop of plain yogurt or coconut cream.

Serves 8 (recipe easily doubles)

How to Bake a Pumpkin: Heat the oven to 350 degrees. Cut a pie pumpkin in half (use a sharp knife and make multiple cuts instead of sawing). Scrape out the gooey insides and save the seeds to make toasted pumpkin seeds (recipe upcoming). Lightly grease a cookie sheet and place the pumpkin flesh-side down. Bake until the pumpkin's skin is lightly browned and the flesh is soft–about 45 – 60 minutes. Let the pumpkin cool. Scoop out the flesh and either puree in a blender or food processor, or mash with a potato masher (a fork can also work). One pie pumpkin usually yields about 3-5 cups of pumpkin puree, although some of the bigger, fleshier ones can yield more. You may also use this method to bake butternut squash or acorn squash although cooking times are less (30 minutes for acorn squash and 45 minutes for butternut squash).

A Note About Coconut Milk: This recipe works great with coconut cream or with any creamy variety of canned coconut milk, usually marketed for Asian or Caribbean cooking (I use my store's brand, but Chaokoh is a good choice with zero oxalate content). Do not use the coconut milks that come in a carton and are marketed as non-dairy milk substitutes (usually are found next to the rice, soy or almond milks). These are too watery and have not been tested for oxalate content.

Holiday Baked Apples

6 large baking apples

2 tablespoons of honey (optional)

6 tablespoons of melted butter or coconut oil

1/2 cup of raisins (optional)

2 tablespoons of pumpkin seeds

1 tablespoon of lemon juice

1 teaspoon of cinnamon

1/2 teaspoon of nutmeg

1 cup of apple cider, water, dark rum or brandy

Preheat the oven to 300 degrees. Peel and core the apples. Pour the melted butter and honey into a small bowl and mix well. Roll each apple in the butter mixture then set the apples in a 9" x 13" baking dish. Reserve the left-over butter mixture. Combine the raisins and pumpkin seeds in a small dish, then stuff the raisin mixture into the hollows of the apples (note: if you have non-low oxalate dieters in the house, you may want to stuff their apples with a raisin/walnut mixture instead). Stir the lemon juice, cinnamon and nutmeg into the left-over butter/honey mixture. Pour as much of this butter mixture into the apple hollows as possible, pouring any left-over into the bottom of the pan. Add the cider to the pan (note: if you use rum or brandy, the alcohol burns off during baking). Bake uncovered until the apples are tender when pierced with a fork (about 1 hour). You do not need to baste these apples. Serve warm with the pan syrup and heavy cream or coconut cream.

Makes 6 servings.

Low Oxalate Info: Holiday Baked Apples have about 5 mg. oxalate each when made with apple cider.   Cinnamon (8.3 mg. per teaspoon) and pumpkin seeds (5.2 mg. per 2 tablespoons) are medium oxalate ingredients. Rum and brandy have not been tested, although all liqueurs, whiskeys and wines tested so far have no oxalate or trace amounts of oxalate, so I feel confident using rum or brandy for special occasion cooking.   All other ingredients are low or very low oxalate.

Best Banana Ice Cream

2 frozen bananas (medium to large)

1/4 cup cold coconut milk

6-8 drops liquid stevia or 1 teaspoon honey (optional)

a pinch of nutmeg (1/8 – 1/4 teaspoon)

Put all of the ingredients in the bowl of your food processor (or in your blender). Let sit for about 10 minutes (time will vary depending on how hard the frozen bananas are and how powerful your food processor is.) Process until smooth.   If the ice cream processes very easily and seems too "melted," then the bananas sat for too long. Try only five minutes next time. If your processor can't process the frozen bananas, even with some pulsing or breaking the bananas apart with a spoon, then you need to let them thaw a little longer. When you reach a creamy, soft-serve ice cream consistency, pour the ice cream into bowls and enjoy!

Makes 3 servings (about a half cup each)

Strawberry Paleo Ice Cream

2 frozen bananas (medium to large)

1/2 cup of frozen strawberries

1/2 dropper liquid stevia or 1 teaspoon honey (optional)

1/4 cup of coconut milk

Put all of the ingredients in the bowl of your food processor (or in your blender). Let sit for about 10 minutes (time will vary depending on how hard the frozen bananas are and how powerful your processor is.) Process until smooth. If the ice cream processes very easily and seems too "melted," then it sat for too long. Try only five minutes next time. If your processor can't process the frozen bananas, even with some pulsing or breaking the bananas apart with a spoon, then you need to let them thaw a little longer. When you reach a creamy, soft-serve ice cream consistency, pour the ice cream into bowls and enjoy.

Makes 4 servings (about a half cup each)

Low Oxalate Info: Strawberry Paleo Ice Cream has about 5 mg. oxalate per half cup serving if you use pure coconut milk without guar gum (see Low Oxalate Info under Best Banana Ice Cream for coconut milk suggestions).

Other Diets: Paleo ice cream may also be appropriate for Paleo, gluten-free, dairy-free, GFCF, GAPS, SCD, vegan and vegetarian diets.

Dips and Appetizers:
Black-Eye Pea Fritters (Akara)
For the Sauce:

1 cup of onions

1 cup of red pepper

1/2 cup of big beef tomatoes

1/8 – 1/2 teaspoon of ground cayenne pepper

Dash of salt
2 T coconut oil or peanut oil

For the Fritters:

1 cup dry black-eye peas (or two cups cooked/canned black-eye peas)

1 teaspoon of apple cider vinegar or lemon juice (if using dry beans)

1/2 cup of minced onion

1/8 – 1/4 teaspoon of cayenne pepper

1/2 teaspoon of salt

6-8 tablespoons of water

coconut oil or peanut oil for pan frying (these are the traditional oils used)

Step 1: Set the dry beans and apple cider vinegar in a large bowl with enough water to cover them by a 3-4 inches. Let the peas soak for 12 -24 hours. Remove any floating "skins" or debris. Drain the peas and rinse.

Step 2: Make the sauce. Puree the onions, red pepper, tomato, cayenne, and salt in a food processor or blender. Warm the oil over medium heat.   Add the puree and cook, stirring occasionally, until most of the liquid is evaporated about 10 – 12 minutes. Note: You can dice the veggies really fine and leave this sauce chunky is you prefer.

Step 3. Put the rinsed black-eye peas, onions and cayenne pepper in a high quality/powerful food processor or a high quality/powerful blender. Pulse until you get something similar to a corn meal consistency – it will still be "grainy'" but shouldn't have big chunks of bean (My Cuisinart Elite Food Processor handles this easily in less than 30 seconds). If you do not have a powerful blender or food processor, you will probably want to use cooked/canned peas to get a smooth consistency. Add the salt and 6 tablespoons of water and mix until well-blended. The batter should drip slowly off a spoon.   If it is too thick add up to 2 tablespoons more water until the right consistency is achieved.

Note: I highly recommend using the soaked dry beans if you have the equipment because the fritters are much easier to cook and have a more pleasant, bread-like texture.   If you use cooked/canned peas, for your black-eye pea fritters you will definitely want to use eggs or corn meal as a binder. You will also need to experiment with the water. These fritters still taste great, but they'll have a creamier consistency that isn't as bread-like as a fritter made with soaked dry beans.

Step 4. Africans traditionally deep fry black-eye pea fritters, but I find you can pan fry them in 1/2 – 1 inch oil with good results. Add about a half inch oil to a heavy skillet or dutch oven over medium to medium-high heat. Test the oil with drops of batter – it should bubble when ready. Drop fritters into the oil by tablespoons (get really close to the oil and ease the batter in to keep it from breaking apart). Fry on each side for about 1.5 to 2 minutes. Drain the black-eye-pea fritters on paper towels, adding more oil as needed. After each batch, use a slotted spoon to scoop out any broken up "extras." These crispies are not only yummy, but if you let them stay in the oil too long they will burn and make all of your later batches taste burnt.

Serve with hot sauce.

Makes 24 – 36 fritters depending on your interpretation of a tablespoon . . .

If Your Batter Breaks Apart While Cooking: Keeping your black-eye pea fritters from falling apart is a learned skill. Easing them into the oil gently (dropping from a half inch above the oil) helps a lot. So does chilling the batter. The real problem for me comes with the flip. Like a pancake, it will work better if you make the fritters small and somewhat flat (so they set most of the way through before the flip). I find using both a metal spatula and a spoon helps me ease the fritters over. If this doesn't work for you and you don't care about being authentic, you may add an egg or two to the batter as a binder. Vegans may add a tablespoon or two of corn meal.

1 ½ cup of garbanzo beans, cooked* (one 15 oz. can, rinsed and drained)

juice of one lemon (about 2 teaspoons)

1/2 tablespoon of olive oil

Salt to taste (try ¼ teaspoon at first)

2-4 garlic cloves, minced

½ cup water

Put about half the garbanzo beans and all the rest of the ingredients in your blender or food processor and blend until smooth and creamy. Slowly add the rest of the garbanzo beans, blending after each addition. If you have trouble blending or the consistency seems too dry, add a little more of the magic hummus ingredient— water! I use up to a cup of water to get a smooth, creamy hummus.

Yield: Makes about 1 cup hummus (this recipe can be doubled easily)

Oxalate Note: Garbanzo beans have 8.4 mg. oxalate per ½ cup and are in the medium group.

Each 1/4 cup serving of medium oxalate hummus has 6.6 mg. oxalate. You may also sprinkle your hummus with paprika (6 mg. oxalate per teaspoon), if you want it to look especially pretty for a special occasion.

Broccoli Beef

2 tablespoons of olive oil, lard or coconut oil {UK readers click here, Canadians here)

5 cloves of garlic, minced

1 tablespoon of raw ginger, minced

1.5 lbs. flank steak, cut against the grain (or just buy stir-fry beef from the meat counter)

3/4 cup onion, course chopped (about 1 medium onion)

3 – 4 cups broccoli florets (1 large head or a 12 – 16 oz. bag, frozen)

1/4 cup of Coconut Aminos

1 tablespoon of sesame oil

1/8 teaspoon of cayenne pepper (optional)

1/2 teaspoon of white pepper

salt to taste

Heat the oil in a large skillet or wok over medium heat. Add the garlic and ginger and stir-fry for 1 minute. Add the meat and stir-fry until browned, about 2-3 minutes. Add the onions and broccoli and continue to stir-fry for 1-2 minutes, stirring often. Add the coconut aminos, sesame oil, cayenne and a pinch or two of white pepper. Continue to stir-fry another 1-3 minutes until the broccoli and onions reach your desired "doneness" and the flavors mix. Adjust the seasonings, salting if desired.

Serve over steamed, long-grain rice or cauliflower rice, or eat it plain, my favorite way.

Makes 6 hearty servings.

Chicken Enchiladas Verde

2 1/2 cups of cooked chicken or turkey, shredded

1/2 cup of sour cream

3 cups of shredded cheese (or use 1 cup cream cheese and 2 cups shredded cheese)

1/4 cup of cilantro

4 – 8 corn tortillas (optional)

1 recipe verde sauce (see below)

olive oil

Step 1: Mix the chicken, sour cream, 2 cups of the cheese, and the cilantro in a large bowl.

Step 2: Heat the oil in a skillet and lightly toast each tortilla until it is soft and pliable.

Step 3: Traditional Enchiladas: (8 tortillas): Pour about 1/2 cup verde sauce in the bottom of a 13 x9 inch baking dish. Put about 1/2 – 2/3 cup of the filling in the middle of each tortilla and try to roll it up. If it's too thick to roll up, then try to cut the tortilla around the filling as much as possible as you place it into the pan.

Enchilada Casserole (4 – 8 tortillas): Pour about 1/2 cup verde sauce in the bottom of a 13 x 9 inch baking dish. Line the bottom of the pan with four tortillas (you may need to overlap a little and cut two of the tortillas in half or thirds). Put the filling over the top of the tortillas. If you want, top with four more tortillas (I usually don't top mine).

Grain-Free Chicken Enchiladas Verde: Follow the directions for the casserole except don't use any tortillas. This works nicely for families where some members eat corn and others don't (or some are on the LOD and others aren't). The ones who eat tortillas can either spoon some of the finished casserole onto a tortilla or eat it like an open-faced enchilada, or they can eat it with tortilla chips.

Step 4: Pour the rest of the verde sauce over the enchilas. Top the enchiladas with the remaining cheese and bake in a 350 degree oven for about 20 – 25 minutes until the enchiladas are bubbly and starting to brown.

Serves 8.

Verde Sauce

2 T olive oil

2 cans (4 ounces) fire-roasted Ortega green chiles, chopped

8-10 cloves garlic

1 cup of onion, chopped

2 T lime juice

2-3 cups of chicken broth or water

1/4 cup of cilantro

1/2 teaspoon of salt (if using water)

Put the oil, chilis, garlic and onion in a sauce pan and saute over medium heat until the onions are just beginning to brown (about 5 minutes.) Put the cooked veggies, lime juice, 2 cups of chicken broth, cilantro and salt into your blender and blend until smooth. Add extra broth as needed to achieve a sauce-like consistency (I like mine on the runny side, so I usually use the full extra cup of broth). Note: If you prefer a "greener" sauce, try adding a little bit of whatever low oxalate green veggie you have hanging around (unpeeled zucchini and fresh basil leaves work nicely.) Just remember this adds a little to the oxalate content.

Makes 3 cups of thick verde sauce or 4 cups of thin verde sauce

Low Oxalate Info: Chicken Enchiladas Verde have 6.5 mg. oxalate per serving when made with 8 tortillas, 5 mg. oxalate per serving when made with 4 tortillas, and 3.5 mg. oxalate per serving when made without tortillas.

 If you choose to skip the enchiladas and use this fabulous sauce to top grilled chicken or fish, make the verde sauce thicker (use only 2 cups broth.) One recipe of verde sauce has 25 mg. oxalate (about 4 mg. oxalate per half cup of thick sauce or about 3.1 mg. oxalate per half cup of thin sauce).

French Beef Stew

2 pounds boneless beef stew meat, cubed (I prefer to eat grassfed, organic or omega 3 meat)

2 cups of dry, red wine

2 tablespoons of olive oil

6 – 8 large cloves garlic

1 bay leaf

1 teaspoon of thyme

1/2 teaspoon of freshly ground black pepper

4-6 ounces of bacon, diced

2 cups of yellow onions, chopped

2 cups of mushrooms, sliced (about 8 ounces)

1/2 teaspoon of Celtic sea salt (or to taste)

Put the first seven ingredients in a covered bowl in the refrigerator for at least one hour, or up to 24 hours, turning the meat occasionally. Drain the beef, reserving the liquid (I do this over a collander). Heat a large dutch oven over medium heat and add the bacon. Cook until the bacon is brown. Remove the bacon, leaving the fat in the pan. Add the beef to the bacon fat and cook until almost browned (if you don't have enough fat, add some olive oil). Add the onions and mushrooms and continue to cook until the beef is browned and the onions are translucent. Stir in the marinade, salt and the bacon and bring to a boil. Reduce the heat to low, and cook covered, until the meat is tender, usually 1 – 1.5 hours. Add salt to taste and cook until the liquid is reduced to whatever consistency you chose. Serve with turnips, butternut squash or cooked greens (kale or collard greens are nice). It's also quite yummy served over the top of mashed cauliflower.

Serves 8

1/2 cup of strawberries

1 T of lemon juice

1/2 tsp of fresh, minced ginger

1/2 pound of ground beef (I prefer grass-fed or omega 3 beef)

pinch of salt

2 T of Sun butter (or other low oxalate sunflower spread)

Place the strawberries, lemon juice and ginger in a small sauce pan or skillet and cook until the strawberries are soft. Mash the cooked strawberries with a fork if you want a jam-like appearance. Meanwhile, shape the ground beef into patties after salting to taste. Grill or fry the patties in a skillet over medium heat. Melt the Sunbutter in the microwave (or a small saucepan) until smooth and creamy. When the patties are brown on both sides, remove from heat and put 1 T of melted Sunbutter on each patty. Add half the strawberry mixture to each patty and serve on a bed of lettuce for a grain-free burger. Alternately, you may wish to serve the burger on a Kinnikinuck Tapioca Rice Hamburger Bun (8.3 mg. oxalate per bun) or Odi's gluten-free sandwich bread (7.1 mg. oxalate per slice).

Makes two quarter pound burgers.

Low Oxalate Info: Sunbutter (6.1 mg. per 2 T) and strawberries (7.8 mg. oxalate per half cup) are medium oxalate. All other ingredients are low oxalate or very low oxalate. Each Sunbutter burger has about 7.5 mg. oxalate when served plain without the bun or lettuce.

Substitutions: You may substitute your favorite jam, preserves or fruit spread (made with low oxalate fruit) in place of the sauteed strawberries. My family's favorites are Polaner All Natural Blueberry Fruit Spread, St. Dalfour Pineapple and Mango all natural Fruit Spread, and Crofter's Organic Strawberry Fruit Spread.

Picky Eater Pleaser: Try making this without the ginger or add a drop or two of liquid Stevia to the sauteed strawberries. One of my sons loves "mommy's cooked strawberries." The other wants to eat it with only the Sunbutter, although last time he asked for a bun. Then he pulled his burger out and ate it plain, followed by his Sunbutter and Jelly Bun!.

Other Diets: Low Oxalate Sunbutter burgers may also be appropriate for low carbohydrate, Paleo, gluten-free and dairy-free diets.

Banana Blueberry Dairy-Free Milkshakes

1 frozen banana

1/2 cup of frozen blueberries

1 cup of coconut milk

1 T honey or 3-4 drops liquid Stevia (optional)

Put all of the ingredients into a food processor or blender and blend until smooth (if your freezer is super cold you may have to let the banana thaw 10-15 minutes before mixing in order for it to blend). Pour into two frosty mugs and enjoy!

Makes two 7-8 ounce milkshakes

Oxalate Note: Bananas are a medium oxalate fruit with 5.3 mg. oxalate per medium banana. All other ingredients are low or very low oxalate. Banana Blueberry Dairy-Free Milkshakes have about 4.5 mg. oxalate per serving.

Substitutions and Variations: You can substitute strawberries for the blueberries (raising the oxalate content to about 6 mg. per shake). You might also wish to add a couple tablespoons rice protein, egg white protein or pea protein powder. DO NOT leave out the banana frozen bananas are what give this shake its thick, creamy texture!

Other Diets: Banana Blueberry Dairy-Free Milkshakes may also be suitable for gluten-free, dairy-free, vegan, vegetarian, Paleo, GAPS, SCD and GFCF diets.

What are your favorite ways to enjoy low oxalate, dairy-free milkshakes? Let us know in the comments section below.

Hot Chocolate Steamer

1 cup of milk

1/4 cup of Torani's SF Chocolate Syrup (or to taste)

Mix the milk and the syrup in a large glass measuring cup. If you have one of those nifty steamer attachments on your coffee or cappuccino maker, then run your hot chocolate through the steamer attachment and enjoy. If you don't have a steamer, you can either warm the milk in the microwave (on high for about a minute) or on the stove top. It won't be as frothy this way, but it will still be yummy!

Serve in a large mug, or divide in half and share with a friend.

Low Oxalate Additions: Add a dollop of whipped cream, a peppermint stick stirrer, or a pinch of mace or cardamom. My boys love the candy canes but I prefer the mace.

Low Oxalate Info: All ingredients in your Hot Chocolate Steamer are low oxalate. Torani's Sugar Free Chocolate Syrup has about 1.4 mg. oxalate per fourth cup, while milk ranges from 0 – 2.9 mg. per cup depending on the brand and how it was processed. So your hot chocolate steamer has about 1.4 -4.3 mg. oxalate if you drink the whole thing.

MAIN DISHES (VEGETARIAN):

Eggs and Peas with Onion Cream Sauce

1 medium white or yellow onion, sliced (about 1/2 cup)

1 cup of water

8 ounces frozen green peas* (about 1 cup)

8 hard-boiled eggs, cooled and shelled

1/2 cup heavy cream, sour cream OR plain yogurt (see note)

1 tablespoon of butter AND one tablespoon cornstarch (optional, see note)

1/2 cup of milk

1/4 teaspoon of freshly ground black pepper

1/2 teaspoon of salt

2-3 ounces of Swiss cheese

Place the sliced onion in a small saucepan with the water, bring to a boil and boil for five minutes until most of the water has evaporated. Meanwhile put the peas in a 2-quart casserole. Slice the hard-boiled eggs and place over the peas. When the onion is tender, place it in a food processor or blender (with left-over water) and puree. Melt the butter in the warm saucepan and add the cornstarch. Mix well and cook for about 10 seconds. Add the cold milk, stir well, and bring the mixture to a boil, stirring often. When the white sauce boils and thickens, add cream, salt, pepper, and onion puree. Stir the sauce well then pour over sliced eggs. Sprinkle the casserole with Swiss cheese, then place it under the broiler for about 3 - 4 minutes until it is browned. Serve immediately.

Yeild: 4 main dish servings or 8 side dish servings

Note: If you don't want to bother making a white sauce, replace the cream with sour cream or plain yogurt, reduce the milk to 1/4 cup, and leave out the butter and cornstarch. When making your sauce, simply mix the sour cream, milk, onion puree, salt and pepper in the warm sauce pan, then pour over the egg mixture. You will have to broil the casserole a little longer, but it's still quite yummy (especially with sour cream) and only a little runny.

*Oxalate Note: Green peas are a "lower medium" oxalate vegetable with 5.7 mg. oxalate per 1/2 cup. All other ingredients are low oxalate or very low oxalate.

Variations: This is also good with steamed asparagus or sauteed mushrooms instead of peas. I haven't tried it with sauteed zucchini yet, but that's next on my list.

Other Diets: This recipe may also be appropriate for gluten-free (make sure the sour cream is GF), vegetarian, and controlled carbohydrate dieters.

Jamaican Rice and Peas

2 cups cooked pigeon peas, black-eyed peas or kidney beans

1 can of unsweetened Coconut Milk (13.5 ounces)

1 cup of water

2 cups of long grain white rice (not instant!)

1 habanero pepper (optional)

1 teaspoon of dried thyme

2-4 cloves of garlic, crushed

sea salt to taste (start with 1/4 teaspoon)

Put all of the ingredients into a saucepan, including the cooking liquid from the beans if possible (should be about 3/4 cup liquid adjust by adding extra water if necessary). Bring to a boil, then simmer until most of the liquid is absorbed and the rice is tender (about 30 minutes). Remove the habanero pepper and serve.

Makes 4 main dish or 8 side dish servings.

Note: Most Jamaican chefs start by cooking raw pigeon peas (which are soupy like non-drained canned beans), then add the other ingredients to the bean pot. This is why I use the cooking liquid in my recipe. It keeps things easy and more authentic tasting. You may like the texture of this dish better, however, if you drain and rinse the beans first, then add an extra 3/4 cup water.

Kohlrabi Risotto
4 cups kohlrabi

7 cups LO chicken or vegetable broth or stock (homemade or Swanson's 100% natural)

3 tablespoons extra virgin olive oil or butter

1/2 cup minced onion

1 1/2 cups short grain white rice, such as arborio (medium grain is okay, but do not use long grain rice!)

1 to 2 garlic cloves, minced

Salt to taste (may not be needed if you use a commercial chicken broth)

1 cup of dry white wine, like pinot grigio or sauvignon blanc

1 teaspoon of freshly ground white pepper

1/2 cup of freshly grated Parmesan cheese

1/4 – 1/2 teaspoon of freshly ground nutmeg (optional)

1 tablespoon of butter (optional)

1. Peel the kohlrabi, making sure to remove the white, fibrous layer just under the skin (i.e. double peel the kohlrabi), and cut into 1/2-inch dice.

2. Put your stock or broth into a saucepan and bring it to a simmer over medium heat, with a ladle nearby or in the pot. Turn the heat down to low. I personally like a rich, homemade meat broths for risotto, although homemade vegetable broth and Swanson's 100% natural chicken broth are okay. If your broth tastes a little weak you may want to add more onions, garlic or pepper (none of these ingredients will substantially raise the oxalate level

of this dish, so don't be shy about adding them if you need to).

3. Heat the olive oil over medium heat in a wide, heavy saucepan or a heavy dutch oven. (It should have heavy sides, too, not just a heavy bottom.) Add the onion and cook gently (sweat) until the onion is just tender, about 2-3 minutes. Do not brown the onion. Add the diced kohlrabi and the garlic and cook, stirring, until the kohlrabi is crisp-tender, about 5 – 10 minutes. I prefer my kohlrabi on the tender side, as opposed to the crisp side, for this dish.

4. Add the rice and stir until the grains separate and begin to crackle. This won't happen if you skimp on the oil. In fact, you may need to add more oil if your onions seemed to have soaked up most of the oil. Add the wine and stir until it has evaporated and been absorbed by the rice. Add the simmering stock, a couple of ladlefuls (about 1/2 cup) at a time. The stock should just cover the rice, and should be gently bubbling. Cook, stirring often, until the stock is just about absorbed. You can tell it's absorbed and you're ready for another ladleful when you stir the rice and the dry bottom of the pot shows for a moment behind the spoon. If it's not ready, you won't see the bottom of the pot, just stock. Add another ladleful or two of stock and continue to cook, adding more stock and stirring

each time the rice has just about absorbed the stock and you start seeing the bottom of the pan. Note: you do not have to stir constantly, but do stir often. When the rice is tender all the way through but still chewy, in about 25 minutes (give or take five minutes), it is done. You probably used about 6 cups of stock to get to this point but may have used all 7. Add the pepper and adjust salt to taste.

5. Add another ladleful of stock to the rice (add a half cup water if you are out of stock). Stir in the Parmesan, the nutmeg if using, and the butter and remove from the heat. The mixture should be creamy (add more stock if it isn't). Serve right away in wide soup bowls or on plates, spreading the risotto in a thin layer rather than a mound.

Yield: Makes 6 large servings or 10 side dish servings.

Vegan Stuffed Red Peppers

1 fennel seed tea bag

1 cup of apple cider

1 cup of long grain white rice

2 teaspoon of dried thyme

1 teaspoon of dried sage

2 T of olive oil

1/2 cup of diced celery

1 cup of diced onions

1 1/2 cups of Granny Smith apples, peeled and finely diced (about 2 apples)

1/2 teaspoon of salt (or to taste)

1 teaspoon of white pepper

1/2 cup of dried cranberries

1/2 cup of pumpkin seeds

6 medium red bell peppers, tops cut off and hollowed

fresh thyme sprigs for garnish (optional)

Preheat your oven to 350 degrees. In a medium saucepan, bring 1 cup water and the apple cider to boil and add the fennel tea bag. Brew the tea for about five minutes, then remove the tea bag. Add the rice, thyme and sage. Cover the pot and return to boiling. Simmer the rice, covered, until all liquid is absorbed (about 20 minutes).

Meanwhile, heat the olive oil in a large skillet over medium heat. Saute the celery, onions, apples, salt and pepper in the hot oil until they are softened (about five minutes). Combine the cooked rice, sauteed vegetables and fruit. Stir in the cranberries and the pumpkin seeds. Spoon the stuffing into the bell peppers, then stand the peppers upright in a baking dish. Put the top back on if desired (or cut it up for a salad).

Bake for 30 – 35 minutes or until the peppers are tender and stuffing in heated through. To serve, garnish with a thyme sprig if desired.

Apple Pineapple Salad

1 1/2 cups of pineapple (or 1 can pineapple tidbits, packed in juice)

3 apples

1 small zucchini (about 1/2 cup when shredded)

1/3 cup of raisins

1 medium carrot, shredded (about 1/2 cup) (see oxalate note)

Chop (or drain) the pineapple, reserving the juice. Peel and core the apples. Remove the ends from the zucchini and peel if desired. Shred the apples and zucchini and place them in a large serving bowl. Add the pineapple and 1/3 cup of reserved juice. Add the raisins and mix well. This is the low oxalate version of Apple Pineapple salad. You may eat the salad immediately or chill and serve it later. The pineapple juice keeps the apples from turning brown too quickly, so this salad can be made a few hours early or enjoyed the next day as a left-over.

For the non-low oxalate dieters in the house (or for those of you who can tolerate a little more oxalate in your diet), add shredded carrot to individual servings for a medium oxalate version of the salad (see oxalate note). Carrots add a pretty color to the salad, making it a lot more attractive for dinner guests (including Grammy and Papa), plus carrots add great nutrients, fiber, and crunch!

Servings: 6 adult servings (varies depending on how big your apples are)

*Raisins may pose a choking hazard for kids under three. Try boiling the raisins in pineapple juice until they plump (3-5 minutes in the microwave) to make them soft enough for a young child to chew.

**Oxalate Note: One half cup raw grated carrots has 15.3 mg. oxalate. When the salad is divided into 6 servings, the carrots add an extra 2.7 mg. oxalate per serving, pushing this version of the salad into the medium oxalate range (5-15 mg. oxalate per 1/2 cup). All other ingredients are low oxalate (less than 5 mg. oxalate per 1/2 cup).

2 cups of chopped cabbage (green or purple)

1 cup of chopped romaine lettuce

1/4 cup of chopped cilantro

1 1/2 of tablespoons lime juice (about the juice of one lime)

1 tablespoon of olive oil

Combine the cabbage, lettuce and cilantro in a serving bowl. In a separate bowl, mix the lime juice and olive oil. Drizzle the lime dressing over the cabbage mixture and toss to coat. Let chill for ten minutes before serving for best results.

Makes 4 servings.

Note: This salad easily doubles, but it does not save well. Don't make more than you think you will eat within 24 hours.

Oxalate Note: One serving of cilantro lime slaw (about 3/4 cup) has about 2.6 mg. oxalate.

Equipment Note: Low oxalate recipes like cilantro lime slaw are a lot faster and easier to make if you have a good quality food processor. I own a Cuisinart Elite Collection 14 cup food processor with three different size bowls for different size jobs OR to make your entire meal without having to wash a prep bowl in between (heh heh, love that reason). I love my Cuisinart Food Processor! It used to take me an hour to do all the chopping and grating. Now it takes about 5 minutes.

Picky Eater Pleaser: Serve small piles of chopped cabbage, romaine and cilantro separately with the lime and oil dressing as a dipping sauce. One of my sons will eat the romaine and cilantro without the dressing. The other is willing to try a little dressing, but doesn't like the lime taste, so I often reduce the lime juice content when making this dressing for the boys (or I let them pick a different dressing for dipping).

Avocado Egg Salad

1 ripe avocado

1 tablespoon of GF prepared yellow mustard or GF Dijon mustard

1/4 teaspoon of ground white pepper

1 tablespoon of lemon juice

5-6 hard-boiled eggs (use 5 if they're extra large)

salt to taste

1 cup of low oxalate greens, such as Romaine or Arugula

Mash the ripe avocado in a bowl with a fork (leave a few chunks if desired). Add the mustard, white pepper, lemon juice and salt and mix well. Chop the eggs (or mash them with a fork) and fold them into the dressing until well-mixed. Serve on a bed of low oxalate greens such as Romaine lettuce or argula.

Makes two servings. Avocado egg salad is best if eaten right away or within 12 hours.

Low Oxalate Info: All ingredients in avocado egg salad are low oxalate. It has about 2 mg. oxalate per serving when made with Romaine lettuce and Dijon Mustard and about 2.8 mg. oxalate per serving when made with yellow mustard and arugula.

Variations: Add a few tablespoons yogurt for a creamier salad. You may also like a few tablespoons of chopped green onions, a clove of crushed garlic, some rich-tasting olive oil, or a tablespoon or two of chopped herbs, such as cilantro or basil.

Sarah's Applesauce

Recipe Summary

Prep:

10 mins

Cook:

20 mins

Total:

30 mins

Servings:

4

Ingredients

- ½ teaspoon of ground cinnamon

- ¾ cup of water

- 4 apples - peeled, cored and chopped

- ¼ cup of white sugar

Add All Ingredients to Shopping List

Directions

Instructions Checklist

• Step 1

In a saucepan, combine apples, water, sugar, and cinnamon. Cover, and cook over medium heat for 15 to 20 minutes, or until apples are soft. Allow to cool, then mash with a fork or potato masher.

Partner Tip

Nutrition Facts

Per Serving:

121 calories; 0.2 g total fat; 0 mg cholesterol; 3 mg sodium. 31.8 g carbohydrates; 0.4 g protein;

Pretzel Turtles

Ingredients

14 m20 servings82 cals

• 20 small mini pretzels

• 20 chocolate covered caramel candies

• 20 pecan halves

• Add all ingredients to list

Directions

1. Preheat oven to 300 degrees F (150 degrees C).

2. Arrange the pretzels in a single layer on a parchment lined cookie sheet. Place one chocolate covered caramel candy on each pretzel.

3. Bake for 4 minutes. While the candy is warm, press a pecan half onto each candy covered pretzel. Cool completely before storing in an airtight container.

Nutrition Facts

Per Serving: 82 calories; 2.2 g fat; 14.1 g carbohydrates;1.7 g protein; < 1 mg cholesterol; 263 mg sodium.

Smooth Sweet Tea

Ingredients

3 h 20 m 8 servings' 73 cals

Direction

- 1 pinch of baking soda

- 2 cups of boiling water

- 6 tea bags

- 3/4 cup of white sugar

- 6 cups of cool water

• Add all ingredients to list

1. Sprinkle a pinch of baking soda into a 64-ounce, heat-proof, glass pitcher. Pour in boiling water, and add tea bags. Cover, and allow to steep for 15 minutes.

2. Remove tea bags, and discard; stir in sugar until dissolved. Pour in cool water, then refrigerate until cold.

Nutrition Facts

Per Serving: 73 calories; 0 g fat; 18.7 g carbohydrates; 0 g protein; 0 mg cholesterol; 41 mg sodium. Full nutrition

Sauteed Apples

Recipe Summary

Prep:

5 mins

Cook:

15 mins

Total:

20 mins

Servings:

8

Yield:

4 cups

Nutrition Info

Ingredients

Original recipe yields 8 servings

Ingredient Checklist

• ¼ cup of butter

• 4 large tart apples - peeled, cored and sliced 1/4 inch thick

• 2 teaspoons of cornstarch

• ½ cup of cold water

• ½ cup of brown sugar

• ½ teaspoon of ground cinnamon

Directions

Instructions Checklist

• Step 1

In a large skillet or saucepan, melt butter over medium heat; add apples. Cook, stirring constantly, until apples are almost tender, about 6 to 7 minutes.

• Step 2

Dissolve cornstarch in water; add to skillet. Stir in brown sugar and cinnamon. Boil for 2 minutes, stirring occasionally. Remove from heat and serve warm.

Nutrition Facts

Per Serving:

143 calories; 5.9 g total fat; 15 mg cholesterol; 45 mg sodium. 24.3 g carbohydrates; 0.4 g protein; Full Nutrition

Delicious Ham and Potato Soup

"This is a delicious recipe for ham and potato soup that a friend gave to me. It is very easy and the great thing about it is that you can add additional ingredients, more ham, potatoes, etc and it still turns out great."

Ingredients

45 m8 servings195 cals

• 3 1/2 cups of peeled and diced potatoes

• 1/3 cup of diced celery

- 1/3 cup of finely chopped onion

- 3/4 cup of diced cooked ham

- 3 1/4 cups of water

- 2 tablespoons of chicken bouillon granules

- 1/2 teaspoon of salt, or to taste

- 1 teaspoon of ground white or black pepper, or to taste

- 5 tablespoons of butter

- 5 tablespoons of all-purpose flour

- 2 cups of milk

- Add all ingredients to list

Directions

- Prep 20 m

- Cook 25 m

- Ready In 45 m

1. Combine the potatoes, celery, onion, ham and water in a stockpot. Bring to a boil, then cook over medium heat until potatoes are tender, about 10 to 15 minutes. Stir in the chicken bouillon, salt and pepper.

2. In a separate saucepan, melt butter over medium-low heat. Whisk in flour with a fork, and cook, stirring constantly until thick, about 1 minute. Slowly stir in milk as not to allow lumps to form until all of the milk has been added. Continue stirring over medium-low heat until thick, 4 to 5 minutes.

3. Stir the milk mixture into the stockpot, and cook soup until heated through. Serve immediately.

Nutrition Facts

Per Serving: 195 calories; 10.5 g fat; 19.5 g carbohydrates; 6.1 g protein; 30 mg cholesterol; 394 mg sodium. Full nutrition

Tasty Collard Greens

A classic recipe for collard greens that uses smoked turkey to add some flavor. Greens are simmered in chicken stock, then spiced with a dash of red chile flakes.

Recipe Summary

Prep: 30 mins

Cook: 2 hrs

Total: 2 hrs 30 mins

Servings: 10

Nutrition Info

Ingredients

Original recipe yields 10 servings

Ingredient Checklist

- ¼ cup of olive oil

- 2 tablespoons minced garlic

- 5 cups of chicken stock

- 1 smoked turkey drumstick

- 5 bunches of collard greens - rinsed, trimmed and chopped

- salt and black pepper to taste

- 1 tablespoon of crushed red pepper flakes (optional)

Directions

Instructions Checklist

- Step 1

Heat olive oil in a large pot over medium heat. Add garlic, and gently saute until light brown. Pour in the chicken stock, and add the turkey leg. Cover the pot, and simmer for 30 minutes.

- Step 2

Add the collard greens to the cooking pot, and turn the heat up to medium-high. Let the greens cook down for about 45 minutes, stirring occasionally.

• Step 3

Reduce heat to medium, and season with salt and pepper to taste. Continue to cook until the greens are tender and dark green, 45 to 60 minutes. Drain greens, reserving liquid. Mix in red pepper flakes if desired. Use liquid to reheat leftovers.

Nutrition Facts

Per Serving:

142 calories; 7.9 g total fat; 23 mg cholesterol; 689 mg sodium. 10.6 g carbohydrates; 9.6 g protein; Full Nutrition

Sausage Stuffed Jalapenos

Recipe Summary

Prep: 25 mins

Cook: 20 mins

Total: 45 mins

Servings: 12

Ingredients

Original recipe yields 12 servings

Ingredient Checklist

• 1 pound of ground pork sausage

• 1 (8 ounce) package of cream cheese, softened

• 1 cup of shredded Parmesan cheese

• 1 pound of large fresh jalapeno peppers, halved lengthwise and seeded

• 1 (8 ounce) bottle Ranch dressing (optional)

Directions

Instructions Checklist

• Step 1

Preheat oven to 425 degrees F (220 degrees C).

• Step 2

Place sausage in a skillet over medium heat, and cook until evenly brown. Drain grease.

• Step 3

In a bowl, mix the sausage, cream cheese, and Parmesan cheese. Spoon about 1 tablespoon sausage mixture into each jalapeno half. Arrange stuffed halves in baking dishes.

• Step 4

Bake 20 minutes in the preheated oven, until bubbly and lightly browned. Serve with Ranch dressing.

Per Serving:

362 calories; 34.3 g total fat; 58 mg cholesterol; 601 mg sodium. 4.3 g carbohydrates; 9.2 g protein; Full Nutrition

Rosemary Roasted Turkey

This recipe makes your turkey moist and full of flavor. You can also use this recipe for Cornish game hens, chicken breasts or roasting chicken. Select a turkey sized according to the amount of people you will be serving."

Ingredients

4 h 45 m 16 servings 596 cals

• 3/4 cup of olive oil

• 3 tablespoons of minced garlic

• 2 tablespoons of chopped fresh rosemary

• 1 tablespoon of chopped fresh basil

• 1 tablespoon of Italian seasoning

• 1 teaspoon of ground black pepper

- salt to taste

- 1 (12 pound) of whole turkey

- Add all ingredients to list

Directions

- Prep 25 m

- Cook 4 h

- Ready In 4 h 45 m

1. Preheat oven to 325 degrees F (165 degrees C).

2. In a small bowl, mix the olive oil, garlic, rosemary, basil, Italian seasoning, black pepper and salt. Set aside.

3. Wash the turkey inside and out; pat dry. Remove any large fat deposits. Loosen the skin from the breast. This is done by slowly working your fingers between the breast and the skin. Work it loose to the end of the drumstick, being careful not to tear the skin.

4. Using your hand, spread a generous amount of the rosemary mixture under the breast skin and down the thigh and leg. Rub the remainder of the rosemary mixture over the outside of the breast. Use toothpicks to seal skin over any exposed breast meat.

5. Place the turkey on a rack in a roasting pan. Add about 1/4 inch of water to the bottom of the pan. Roast in the preheated oven 3 to 4 hours, or until the internal temperature of the bird reaches 180 degrees F (80 degrees C).

Nutrition Facts

Per Serving: 596 calories; 33.7 g fat; 0.8 g carbohydrates;68.1 g protein; 198 mg cholesterol; 165 mg sodium. Full nutrition

Best Lemonade Ever

Ingredients

4 h 35 m 10 servings 145 cals

- 1 3/4 cups of white sugar

- 8 cups of water

- 1 1/2 cups of lemon juice

- Add all ingredients to list

Directions

- Prep 30 m

- Cook 5 m

- Ready In 4 h 35 m

1. In a small saucepan, combine sugar and 1 cup water. Bring to boil and stir to dissolve sugar. Allow to cool to room temperature, then cover and refrigerate until chilled.

2. Remove seeds from lemon juice, but leave pulp. In pitcher, stir together chilled syrup, lemon juice and remaining 7 cups water.

Nutrition Facts

Per Serving: 145 calories; 0 g fat; 38.2 g carbohydrates;0.1 g protein; 0 mg cholesterol; 6 mg sodium. Full nutrition

Luscious Slush Punch

"This is without a doubt the best punch I've ever had! Makes enough for 2 punch bowls. This is our Christmas Eve punch tradition, and there is never a drop left!"

Ingredients

8 h 20 m 50 servings 108 cals

- 2 1/2 cups white sugar

- 6 cups of water

- 2 (3 ounce) packages of strawberry flavored Jell-O® mix

- 1 (46 fluid ounce) can pineapple juice

- 2/3 cups of lemon juice

- 1 quart of orange juice

- 2 (2 liter) bottles lemon-lime flavored carbonated beverage

- Add all ingredients to list

Directions

- Prep 15 m

- Cook 5 m

- Ready In 8 h 20 m

1. Bring the sugar, water, and strawberry flavored gelatin to a boil in a large saucepan; boil for 3 minutes. Stir in the pineapple juice, lemon juice, and orange juice. Divide mixture into 2 separate containers and freeze.

2. Combine the contents of 1 container with 1 bottle of the lemon-lime flavored carbonated beverage in a punch bowl; stir until slushy. Repeat with remaining portions as needed.

Nutrition Facts

Per Serving: 108 calories; 0.1 g fat; 27.4 g carbohydrates;0.6 g protein; 0 mg cholesterol; 25 mg sodium. Full nutrition

Ingredients

5 h 10 m 16 servings 545 cals

- 1 (12 pound) of whole turkey

- 6 tablespoons of butter, divided

- 4 cups of warm water

- 3 tablespoons of chicken bouillon

- 2 tablespoons of dried parsley

- 2 tablespoons of dried minced onion

- 2 tablespoons of seasoning salt

- Add all ingredients to list

Directions

Add a notePrint

- Prep 10 m

- Cook 5 h

- Ready In 5 h 10 m

1. Preheat oven to 350 degrees F (175 degrees C). Rinse and wash turkey. Discard the giblets, or add to pan if they are anyone's favorites.

2. Place turkey in a Dutch oven or roasting pan. Separate the skin over the breast to make little

pockets. Put 3 tablespoons of the butter on both sides between the skin and breast meat. This makes for very juicy breast meat.

3. In a medium bowl, combine the water with the bouillon. Sprinkle in the parsley and minced onion. Pour over the top of the turkey. Sprinkle seasoning salt over the turkey.

4. Cover with foil, and bake in the preheated oven 3 1/2 to 4 hours, until the internal temperature of the turkey reaches 180 degrees F (80 degrees C). For the last 45 minutes or so, remove the foil so the turkey will brown nicely.

Nutrition Facts

Per Serving: 545 calories; 27.9 g fat; 0.9 g carbohydrates;68.1 g protein; 210 mg cholesterol; 560 mg sodium.

Big Al's K.C. Bar-B-Q Sauce
Ingredients

35 m 48 servings 46 cals

• 2 cups of ketchup

• 2 cups of tomato sauce

• 1 1/4 cups of brown sugar

• 1 1/4 cups of red wine vinegar

- 1/2 cup of unsulfured molasses

- 4 teaspoons of hickory-flavored liquid smoke

- 2 tablespoons of butter

- 1/2 teaspoon of garlic powder

- 1/2 teaspoon of onion powder

- 1/4 teaspoon of chili powder

- 1 teaspoon of paprika

- 1/2 teaspoon of celery seed

- 1/4 teaspoon of ground cinnamon

- 1/2 teaspoon of cayenne pepper

- 1 teaspoon of salt

- 1 teaspoon of coarsely ground black pepper

- Add all ingredients to list

Directions

- Prep 15 m

- Cook 20 m

- Ready In 35 m

1. In a large saucepan over medium heat, mix together the ketchup, tomato sauce, brown sugar, wine vinegar, molasses, liquid smoke and butter. Season with garlic powder, onion powder, chili

powder, paprika, celery seed, cinnamon, cayenne, salt and pepper.

2. Reduce heat to low, and simmer for up to 20 minutes. For thicker sauce, simmer longer, and for thinner, less time is needed. Sauce can also be thinned using a bit of water if necessary. Brush sauce onto any kind of meat during the last 10 minutes of cooking.

Nutrition Facts

Per Serving: 46 calories; 0.9 g fat; 9.9 g carbohydrates;0.3 g protein; 1 mg cholesterol; 219 mg sodium. Full nutrition

Southern Pimento Cheese

Recipe Summary

Prep: 10 mins

Total: 10 mins

Servings: 12

Yield: 3 cups

Ingredients

Original recipe yields 12 servings

Ingredient Checklist

- 2 cups of shredded extra-sharp Cheddar cheese

- 8 ounces of cream cheese, softened

- ½ cup of mayonnaise

- ¼ teaspoon of garlic powder

- ¼ teaspoon of ground cayenne pepper (optional)

- ¼ teaspoon of onion powder

- 1 jalapeno pepper, seeded and minced (optional)

- 1 (4 ounce) jar diced pimento, drained

- salt and black pepper to taste

Directions

Instructions Checklist

- Step 1

Place the Cheddar cheese, cream cheese, mayonnaise, garlic powder, cayenne pepper, onion powder, minced jalapeno, and pimento into the large bowl of a mixer. Beat at medium speed, with paddle if possible, until thoroughly combined. Season to taste with salt and black pepper.

Nutrition Facts

Per Serving:

208 calories; 19.9 g total fat; 44 mg cholesterol; 229 mg sodium. 2.1 g carbohydrates; 6.3 g protein; Full Nutrition

Guacamole

Recipe Summary

Prep: 10 mins

Total: 10 mins

Servings: 4

Ingredients

Ingredient Checklist

• 3 avocados - peeled, pitted, and mashed

• 1 lime, juiced

• 1 teaspoon of salt

• ½ cup of diced onion

• 3 tablespoons of chopped fresh cilantro

• 2 roma (plum) tomatoes, diced

• 1 teaspoon of minced garlic

• 1 pinch of ground cayenne pepper (optional)

Add All Ingredients to Shopping List

Directions

Instructions Checklist

• Step 1

In a medium bowl, mash together the avocados, lime juice, and salt. Mix in onion, cilantro, tomatoes, and garlic. Stir in cayenne pepper. Refrigerate 1 hour for best flavor, or serve immediately.

Tips

Upgrade your cutting boards using our guide to the best cutting boards on the market, then use them to prepare our favorite recipes.

Nutrition Facts

Per Serving:

262 calories; 22.2 g total fat; 0 mg cholesterol; 596 mg sodium. 18 g carbohydrates; 3.7 g protein; Full Nutrition

Grilled Asparagus

Recipe Summary

Prep: 15 mins

Cook: 3 mins

Total: 18 mins

Servings: 4

Ingredient Checklist

- 1 pound of fresh asparagus spears, trimmed

- 1 tablespoon of olive oil

- Salt and pepper to taste

Directions

Instructions Checklist

- Step 1

Preheat grill for high heat.

- Step 2

Lightly coat the asparagus spears with olive oil. Season with salt and pepper to taste.

- Step 3

Grill over high heat for 2 to 3 minutes, or to desired tenderness.

Nutrition Facts

Per Serving:

53 calories; 3.5 g total fat; 0 mg cholesterol; 2 mg sodium. 4.4 g carbohydrates; 2.5 g protein; Full Nutrition

Recipe Summary

Prep: 30 mins

Cook: 10 mins

Total: 2 hrs 40 mins

Additional: 2 hrs

Servings: 6

Ingredient Checklist

- 1 cup of olive oil

- ¼ cup of chopped fresh parsley

- 1 lemon, juiced

- 2 tablespoons of hot pepper sauce

- 3 cloves of garlic, minced

- 1 tablespoon of tomato paste

- 2 teaspoons of dried oregano

- 1 teaspoon of salt

- 1 teaspoon of ground black pepper

- 2 pounds of large shrimp, peeled and deveined with tails attached

- Skewers

Directions

Instructions Checklist

• Step 1

In a mixing bowl, mix together olive oil, parsley, lemon juice, hot sauce, garlic, tomato paste, oregano, salt, and black pepper. Reserve a small amount for basting later. Pour remaining marinade into a large resealable plastic bag with shrimp. Seal, and marinate in the refrigerator for 2 hours.

• Step 2

Preheat grill for medium-low heat. Thread shrimp onto skewers, piercing once near the tail and once near the head. Discard marinade.

• Step 3

Lightly oil grill grate. Cook shrimp for 5 minutes per side, or until opaque, basting frequently with reserved marinade.

Note

The nutrition data for this recipe includes information for the full amount of the marinade ingredients. Depending on marinating time, ingredients, cooking method, etc., the actual amount of the marinade consumed will vary.

Nutrition Facts

Per Serving:

447 calories; 37.5 g total fat; 230 mg cholesterol; 800 mg sodium. 3.7 g carbohydrates; 25.3 g protein; Full Nutrition

Jamie's Sweet and Easy Corn on the Cob

Recipe Summary

Prep: 5 mins

Cook: 10 mins

Total: 15 mins

Servings: 6

Ingredient Checklist

- 2 tablespoons of white sugar

- 1 tablespoon of lemon juice

- 6 ears corn on the cob, husks and silk removed

Directions

- Step 1

Fill a large pot about 3/4 full of water and bring to a boil. Stir in sugar and lemon juice, dissolving the sugar. Gently place ears of corn into boiling water, cover the pot, turn off the heat, and let the corn cook in the hot water until tender, about 10 minutes.

Nutrition Facts

Per Serving:

94 calories; 1.1 g total fat; 0 mg cholesterol; 14 mg sodium. 21.5 g carbohydrates; 2.9 g protein; Full Nutrition

Roasted Rack of Lamb
Ingredients

40 m 4 servings 481 cals

- 1/2 cup of fresh bread crumbs

- 2 tablespoons of minced garlic

- 2 tablespoons of chopped fresh rosemary

- 1 teaspoon of salt

- 1/4 teaspoon of black pepper

- 2 tablespoons of olive oil

- 1 (7 bone) rack of lamb, trimmed and frenched

- 1 teaspoon of salt

- 1 teaspoon of black pepper

- 2 tablespoons of olive oil

• 1 tablespoon of Dijon mustard

• Add all ingredients to list

Directions

• Prep 20 m

• Cook 20 m

• Ready In 40 m

1. Preheat oven to 450 degrees F (230 degrees C). Move oven rack to the center position.

2. In a large bowl, combine bread crumbs, garlic, rosemary, 1 teaspoon salt and 1/4 teaspoon pepper. Toss in 2 tablespoons olive oil to moisten mixture. Set aside.

3. Season the rack all over with salt and pepper. Heat 2 tablespoons olive oil in a large heavy oven proof skillet over high heat. Sear rack of lamb for 1 to 2 minutes on all sides. Set aside for a few minutes. Brush rack of lamb with the mustard. Roll in the bread crumb mixture until evenly coated. Cover the ends of the bones with foil to prevent charring.

4. Arrange the rack bone side down in the skillet. Roast the lamb in preheated oven for 12 to 18 minutes, depending on the degree of doneness you want. With a meat thermometer, take a reading in the center of the meat after 10 to 12 minutes and

remove the meat, or let it cook longer, to your taste. Let it rest for 5 to 7 minutes, loosely covered, before carving between the ribs.

Note

• Allow internal temperature to be 5 to 10 degrees less than you like because the meat will continue to cook while it sits. Bloody rare: 115 to 125 degrees F Rare: 125 to 130 degrees F Medium rare: 130 to 140 degrees F Medium: 140 to 150 degrees F

• Partner Tip

• Reynolds Aluminum foil can be used to keep food moist, cook it evenly, and make clean-up easier.

Nutrition Facts

Per Serving: 481 calories; 40.8 g fat; 5.6 g carbohydrates;22.2 g protein; 94 mg cholesterol; 1369 mg sodium. Full nutrition

Recipe Summary

Prep: 20 mins

Cook: 40 mins

Total: 2 hrs 30 mins

Additional: hr 30 mins

Servings: 24

Yield: 2 - 9x5 inch loaves

Ingredient Checklist

• 2 cups of warm water (110 degrees F/45 degrees C)

• ⅔ cup of white sugar

• 1 ½ tablespoons of active dry yeast

• 1 ½ teaspoons of salt

• ¼ cup of vegetable oil

• 6 cups of bread flour

Directions

Instructions Checklist

• Step 1

In a large bowl, dissolve the sugar in warm water, and then stir in yeast. Allow to proof until yeast resembles a creamy foam.

• Step 2

Mix salt and oil into the yeast. Mix in flour one cup at a time. Knead dough on a lightly floured surface until smooth. Place in a well oiled bowl, and turn dough to coat. Cover with a damp cloth. Allow to rise until doubled in bulk, about 1 hour.

• Step 3

Punch dough down. Knead for a few minutes, and divide in half. Shape into loaves, and place into two well oiled 9x5 inch loaf pans. Allow to rise for 30 minutes, or until dough has risen 1 inch above pans.

•s Step 4

Bake at 350 degrees F (175 degrees C) for 30 minutes.

Nutrition Facts

Per Serving:

168 calories; 2.9 g total fat; 0 mg cholesterol; 147 mg sodium. 30.7 g carbohydrates; 4.4 g protein;

Low oxalate snacks

These foods are quite useful for busy people who wish to follow a strict low oxalate diet. Here are some great ideas on the same.

No-bake bars

These snacks are ideal for anyone looking to get a protein boost as you go about your activities. This recipe serves nine people, and it requires the following ingredients:

• 2 cups of oats

• Three tablespoons of unsweetened coconut shreds

• One large ripe banana

• One tablespoon of milled flaxseed

• Three scoops of vanilla protein powder

• ½ a cup of sunflower butter

• ½ a cup of melted coconut oil

Directions

Start by mashing the ripe banana and when it forms a smooth consistency, proceed to add all the other ingredients. Press the mixture onto a square pan before setting it in a freezer for at least thirty minutes. From here, you can work on cutting it into squares which you can then wrap individually. It is a straightforward recipe, and you should finish making the bars within an hour.

Coconut flour cookies

It is quite a hassle to find a flour that is low in oxalates and coconut flour provides a healthy alternative to the same. The great thing about it is that it also falls in line with other meal plans such as the Paleo diet. The cookies presented below are very easy to make, and you will love how delicious they are. To make them, you will need:

• Three tablespoons of coconut flour

• A tablespoon of honey

• Two tablespoons of cold butter

Directions

You should begin by heating your oven to 365 degrees Fahrenheit. When it comes to baking, I find that adequate preheating ensures that you can finish making your cookies on time and that the hue will be even. From here, you can combine the ingredients. You can choose to do this by hand.

However, you will get the best results if you decide to use a pastry blender or a food processor. Once the ingredients have combined evenly, proceed to divide them into small balls which you will then flatten on a baking sheet. Insert the cookie baking sheet in the oven and let the dough cook for at least nine minutes. Switch off the oven heat and leave the cookies in the oven for two minutes before moving them to a cooling rack.

These wraps are great snacks to have by your side as you move from one activity to the other. You can make a large batch at the beginning of the week to enable you to have an ample supply of these healthy treats. The recipe I have serves four people, and you are free to tweak it to be for as many people as you would prefer. Here is what you need for this:

• Ten cherry tomatoes

• 1 cup of shredded cheddar cheese

• 1 pound of thick bacon

• ½ head butter lettuce

For the bacon, ensure that you cut it into one-inch pieces to make the cooking easy.

Directions

Start by cooking the cut bacon in a large skillet. Ensure that it turns brown on all sides before draining it and placing it on the side. Next, halve the cherry tomatoes. For each lettuce leaf, add ¼ cup of cheddar cheese and add ¼ of the bacon and cherry tomatoes on top. You can then roll up the wraps before cutting them in half.

There are some fruits which you should not eat if you wish to keep kidney stones at bay. That is not to say that you cannot enjoy a delicious bowl of fruit now and then. All you need are low-oxalate fruits cut into large chunks. Place these in a bowl and add a plastic fork and you are set to go to your meetings, and when the hunger pangs strike, you will have the right snack with which to fight them. Here are some fruits that you can consider for a salad: blueberries, pears, apples, and bananas. You should stay away from high-oxalate fruits such as raspberries, kiwis and oranges.

Low oxalate breakfast ideas

Following a low-oxalate diet requires that you take note of what you are eating from when you wake up till the moment you retire to bed. It is essential that you pay close attention to your breakfast given that it is the most important meal of the day. Here are some fun ideas on the same:

Banana Muffins

Bananas are low-oxalate fruits and are thus an excellent choice for use in flavoring muffins. My recipe calls for coconut flour which is also low in oxalates, thus making these muffins a healthy choice. You require:

• Four lightly beaten eggs

- Four mashed ripe bananas

- Two tablespoons of vanilla extract

- Three tablespoons of maple syrup

- ½ a teaspoon of salt

- One teaspoon of baking powder

- ½ a cup of coconut flour

- ½ a teaspoon of baking soda

Directions

Begin by heating your oven to 325 degrees Fahrenheit before embarking on greasing your muffin tins. Next, mix eggs, vanilla extract, banana and maple syrup in a bowl until they are evenly combined. In a separate bowl, add the coconut flour, baking soda, baking powder, and salt and mix them until combined. Pour the dry components to the wet mixture and stir them until they combine evenly.

Let the dough sit outside for at least five minutes before dividing it into the muffin tins. Place the muffin tins into the oven and let them cook for at least twenty minutes. Keep checking to ensure that they do not burn and perform a clean test to see if they are ready.

The rule to this recipe is that you should not exceed one serving if you wish to keep your oxalate levels in check. The reason behind this is that though food may be low in oxalates, having an excess of the meal will add on to the number of oxalates that you are having and will thus put you at risk of having too many oxalates in your system. As such, it is advisable to think of oxalates concentration in a per serving basis as this will help you estimate how much you are taking.

Here is what you need:

• 1 cup of creamy milk

• Two small bananas

• ½ a cup of yogurt

Ensure that the dairy options you choose are non-fat. The bananas can either be frozen or chopped into small pieces.

Directions

Prepare your ingredients and place them in a bar mix or a blender. In a few minutes, your smoothie will be ready, and you will have the energy you need to face the day ahead.

You pay a lot of attention to which nutrients you put into your body for optimal fuel. But what if some of your go-to superfoods (think: berries, nuts, and spinach) contain compounds that not only sabotage some of your nutritional intake, but may also raise your risk for painful, race-stopping kidney stones? This can translate into the question: Is a low-oxalate diet for you?

Yes, it's a real thing. Oxalates belong to a category of compounds dubbed "anti-nutrients" that block the absorption of nutrients. And unfortunately, they're found in highly nutritious foods that probably make a regular appearance on your plate.

While eating an oxalate-rich diet may increase your likelihood of developing calcium oxalate kidney stones, it depends greatly on other factors, including what other foods are in your diet and your hydration status. Other risk factors include certain rare medical conditions like Dent Disease, and Inflammatory Bowel Disease like Crohn's or ulcerative colitis.

The only true way to know if you have high levels of oxalates is through a urine test carried out by your healthcare provider. If your doctor does identify you as having a high risk for the formation of calcium oxalate kidney stones, here's the good news: While you may need to limit high-oxalate foods in your diet, you don't have to avoid them altogether or miss out on all the other good-for-you nutrients they offer.